# CONTENTS

# INTRODUCTION

Welcome to Lean and Green, In a world where our dietary choices impact not only our health but also the well-being of our planet, this book aims to be your guide to a more conscious and fulfilling culinary journey. By marrying the principles of lean eating and sustainable practices, we embark on a delicious adventure that nourishes both body and environment.

In recent years, the concepts of "lean" and "green" have gained significant momentum as individuals seek ways to improve their health while minimizing their ecological footprint. Lean cooking emphasizes the importance of nutrition, portion control, and reducing unnecessary ingredients, while green living encourages us to adopt practices that support the long-term health of our planet.

Within these pages, you will find a diverse collection of recipes that exemplify the harmony between flavor, nutrition, and sustainability. Whether you are a seasoned chef or a kitchen novice, this book offers something for everyone. From vibrant salads bursting with fresh, locally sourced produce to hearty plant-based dishes that celebrate the bounties of nature, each recipe is thoughtfully crafted to deliver wholesome and satisfying meals.

But "Lean and Green" is more than just a cookbook. It is a call to action—a way to reimagine our relationship with food and the environment. As we delve into the world of lean and green cooking, we will explore the interconnectedness between our dietary choices and the planet's well-being. We will learn how simple shifts in our cooking and shopping habits can lead to significant reductions in waste, energy consumption, and greenhouse gas emissions.

Moreover, this book will provide you with practical tips and insights on how to navigate the challenges and hurdles often associated with sustainable cooking. We will explore the importance of mindful meal planning, effective ingredient substitutions, and creative ways to repurpose leftovers, all with the aim of minimizing waste and maximizing flavor.

Beyond the kitchen, we will delve into broader topics

such as the benefits of supporting local farmers and producers, the significance of organic and ethically sourced ingredients, and the potential of incorporating more plant-based meals into our diets. By embracing these practices, we can make a tangible difference in our own lives and contribute to the preservation of our planet's precious resources.

So, whether you are seeking to improve your health, reduce your environmental impact, or simply explore new culinary horizons, "Lean and Green: A Cookbook for Sustainable Living" is here to inspire and empower you. It is an invitation to embark on a culinary adventure that not only delights your taste buds but also leaves a positive mark on our world.

Together, let us savor the joy of cooking and eating in a way that nourishes our bodies, respects the Earth, and sets the stage for a healthier and more sustainable future. Let the journey begin!

# CHAPTER ONE

## Introduction to Lean and Green Eating

### Understanding the principles of lean and green eating

Lean and green eating is a dietary approach that focuses on consuming foods that are both healthy and environmentally friendly. It involves choosing foods that are low in calories and unhealthy fats while also considering their ecological impact. By understanding the principles of lean and green eating, individuals can make informed choices that benefit both their health and the planet.

To better grasp the concept of lean and green eating, let's break down its key principles:

- Minimizing processed foods: Lean and green eating encourages the consumption of whole, unprocessed foods. This means opting for fresh fruits and vegetables, whole grains, lean proteins, and healthy fats instead of packaged and heavily processed foods that are often high in added sugars, unhealthy fats, and preservatives.
- Prioritizing plant-based options: Plants require

fewer resources and generate fewer greenhouse gas emissions compared to animal-based products. Therefore, lean and green eating emphasizes incorporating a variety of fruits, vegetables, legumes, nuts, and seeds into the diet. Plant-based proteins such as tofu, tempeh, and beans can be excellent alternatives to animal-based proteins.

- Choosing sustainable protein sources: When lean and green eating incorporates animal-based proteins, it promotes selecting sustainable sources. This includes opting for seafood that is low in mercury and sustainably caught, as well as poultry and eggs from organic and ethically raised animals. Reducing the consumption of beef and pork, which have a higher environmental impact, is also encouraged.

- Reducing food waste: Lean and green eating emphasizes the importance of minimizing food waste. This can be achieved by planning meals, properly storing perishable foods, and repurposing leftovers. By reducing food waste, individuals not only contribute to environmental sustainability but also save money and resources.

- Considering food packaging: Packaging waste contributes significantly to environmental pollution. Lean and green eating encourages choosing foods with minimal packaging, opting for reusable or recyclable packaging, and supporting local farmers' markets or bulk stores where packaging waste is reduced.

By adhering to these principles, individuals can make

conscious choices that support both personal health and the environment. The next section will delve into the benefits of incorporating lean and green practices into your diet.

## Benefits of incorporating lean and green practices into your diet

Incorporating lean and green practices into your diet can yield numerous benefits, ranging from improved personal health to reduced environmental impact. Here are some key advantages:

- Healthier lifestyle: Lean and green eating promotes the consumption of nutrient-dense foods, such as fruits, vegetables, and whole grains. These foods are rich in vitamins, minerals, and antioxidants, which support overall health and help prevent chronic diseases like heart disease, diabetes, and certain types of cancer. By adopting lean and green practices, individuals can enjoy improved energy levels, enhanced digestion, and better weight management.
- Weight management: Lean and green eating encourages portion control and selecting foods that are low in calories and unhealthy fats. This approach can contribute to weight loss or maintenance goals. Moreover, by prioritizing whole, unprocessed foods, individuals often feel

more satiated and are less likely to overeat.

- Reduced environmental impact: Food production and agriculture contribute significantly to greenhouse gas emissions, deforestation, and water pollution. By following lean and green practices, individuals can decrease their carbon footprint and contribute to environmental sustainability. Choosing plant-based options and sustainable protein sources reduces the strain on natural resources, minimizes habitat destruction, and helps combat climate change.
- Enhanced biodiversity: By consuming a diverse range of plant-based foods, individuals support biodiversity. The cultivation of a variety of crops reduces the need for monoculture farming, which can deplete the soil, require excessive water usage, and contribute to the loss of plant and animal species. Additionally, lean and green practices often involve supporting local farmers and purchasing seasonal produce, which helps preserve traditional farming methods and local ecosystems.
- Financial savings: Lean and green eating can be cost-effective in the long run. By focusing on whole foods and reducing reliance on processed and packaged items, individuals can save money on groceries. Additionally, planning meals, repurposing leftovers, and minimizing food waste can lead to significant financial savings over time.

In summary, incorporating lean and green practices into your diet can lead to improved personal health, reduced environmental impact, enhanced biodiversity, and financial savings. By making conscious food choices, individuals can contribute to their own well-being and the sustainability of the planet.

## The environmental impact of food choices

The environmental impact of our food choices is a significant and often overlooked aspect of our daily lives. From the production and transportation of food to its disposal, every step in the food system has consequences for the environment. Understanding the environmental impact of our food choices is essential for making sustainable decisions and mitigating the negative effects on the pchoice

Here are key factors that contribute to the environmental impact of food choices:

- Greenhouse gas emissions: Food production, particularly the rearing of livestock, is a major contributor to greenhouse gas emissions. The livestock sector alone is responsible for approximately 14.5% of global greenhouse gas emissions, primarily through methane released during enteric fermentation and manure management. Additionally, the use of synthetic fertilizers in agriculture releases nitrous oxide, a potent greenhouse gas.

- Land and water use: The production of food requires vast amounts of land and water resources. Deforestation for agricultural expansion, such as clearing forests for cattle ranching or palm oil plantations, contributes to habitat loss and biodiversity decline. Furthermore, irrigation for crop cultivation can deplete freshwater sources and disrupt ecosystems.
- Energy consumption: Food production, processing, and transportation rely on fossil fuels, contributing to energy consumption and associated carbon emissions. Long-distance transportation of food, especially when shipped by air, generates more emissions compared to locally sourced options. Processing and packaging food also require energy, often derived from non-renewable sources.
- Pesticides and fertilizers: The use of pesticides and synthetic fertilizers in conventional agriculture can have adverse effects on the environment. Pesticides contaminate soil, waterways, and ecosystems, affecting biodiversity and harming beneficial insects. Runoff from fertilizers contributes to water pollution and eutrophication, leading to the formation of harmful algal blooms.
- Food waste: Food waste is a significant environmental issue. When food is wasted, all the resources used in its production, including water, energy, and land, are also wasted. Additionally,

decomposing food in landfills produces methane, a potent greenhouse gas. Reducing food waste is crucial for minimizing the environmental impact of the food system.

By considering these factors and making informed choices, individuals can reduce the environmental impact of their food consumption. The next section will explore how to make sustainable and health-conscious food choices.

## How to make sustainable and health-conscious food choices

Making sustainable and health-conscious food choices requires a combination of knowledge, planning, and mindful decision-making. By following these guidelines, individuals can adopt a more environmentally friendly and healthful approach to their diet:

- Choose whole, unprocessed foods: Base your meals around whole foods such as fruits, vegetables, whole grains, legumes, and nuts. These foods are nutrient-dense and generally have a lower environmental impact compared to processed and packaged alternatives.
- Prioritize plant-based options: Incorporate more plant-based meals into your diet. Opt for plant-based proteins like beans, lentils, tofu, and tempeh instead of meat. Increase your intake of

fruits and vegetables, aiming for a diverse range of colors to obtain a wide array of nutrients.

- Select sustainable protein sources: When consuming animal-based products, choose sustainably sourced options. Look for seafood certified by sustainable seafood organizations, opt for organic and pasture-raised poultry and eggs, and reduce the consumption of beef and pork, which have higher environmental impacts.
- Buy local and seasonal produce: Support local farmers and reduce the carbon footprint associated with long-distance transportation by purchasing locally grown foods. Choose seasonal produce, as it requires fewer resources for cultivation and tends to have better flavor and nutritional value.
- Minimize food waste: Plan your meals, create shopping lists, and store perishable items properly to minimize food waste. Use leftovers creatively and freeze excess food for future use. Compost food scraps to divert them from landfills and contribute to nutrient-rich soil.
- Consider packaging: Opt for foods with minimal packaging or choose products packaged in recyclable or compostable materials. Buy in bulk when possible to reduce packaging waste. Remember to bring reusable bags and containers when shopping to minimize single-use plastic waste.
- Support sustainable farming practices: Look for organic, regenerative, or permaculture-certified products. These farming methods prioritize soil health, biodiversity, and ecological sustainability.

- Stay informed: Educate yourself about the environmental impact of different foods and food production methods. Stay updated on sustainable food practices and initiatives. Engage with local communities and organizations that promote sustainable and ethical food systems.

By adopting these practices, individuals can contribute to a healthier planet while also enjoying the benefits of a nutritious diet. Making sustainable and health-conscious food choices is a continuous journey that requires ongoing learning and adaptation, but the positive impact is well worth the effort.

## Building a Lean and Green Kitchen

### Stocking a sustainable pantry

Stocking a sustainable pantry involves making conscious choices about the food products you purchase and consume regularly. By selecting sustainable options, you can contribute to environmental preservation and support ethical and responsible food production. Here are some key considerations when stocking a sustainable pantry:

- Choose organic and locally sourced products: Look for organic options to minimize exposure to pesticides and support farming practices that prioritize soil health and biodiversity. Additionally, opt for locally sourced products whenever possible to reduce the carbon footprint associated with long-distance transportation.

- Purchase in bulk: Buying pantry staples in bulk reduces packaging waste and often leads to cost savings. Look for stores that offer bulk bins for items like grains, legumes, nuts, and dried fruits. Bring your own reusable containers to fill, minimizing the need for single-use packaging.
- Select sustainable packaging: When choosing packaged products, prioritize those with eco-friendly packaging. Look for items packaged in recyclable or compostable materials. Avoid excessive plastic packaging and opt for glass, paper, or other sustainable alternatives.
- Support fair trade and ethically sourced products: Look for fair trade certifications on items like coffee, tea, chocolate, and spices. Fair trade ensures that producers receive fair wages and work under safe and ethical conditions.
- Reduce processed and packaged foods: Processed and packaged foods often come with excessive packaging, additives, and preservatives. Opt for whole, unprocessed foods whenever possible, as they are healthier and typically have a lower environmental impact.
- Choose sustainable seafood: Seafood is a valuable protein source, but overfishing and destructive fishing practices can harm marine ecosystems. Consult sustainable seafood guides or choose seafood with certifications such as MSC (Marine Stewardship Council) or ASC (Aquaculture

Stewardship Council) to ensure your seafood choices are environmentally responsible.

By stocking your pantry with sustainable options, you contribute to a healthier planet and support ethical and responsible food production practices.

**Essential tools and equipment for a green kitchen**

Equipping your kitchen with essential tools and equipment that promote sustainability and energy efficiency can help reduce your environmental impact. Here are some key items for a green kitchen:

- Energy-efficient appliances: When purchasing kitchen appliances, look for energy-efficient models. Energy Star-certified appliances, such as refrigerators, dishwashers, and ovens, are designed to consume less energy while still performing effectively.
- Induction cooktops: Induction cooktops use electromagnetic technology to heat pans directly, resulting in faster and more energy-efficient cooking. Compared to traditional gas or electric stovetops, induction cooktops waste less heat and are safer to use.
- High-quality knives and cookware: Investing in high-quality knives and cookware ensures they last longer and reduces the need for frequent replacements. Choose durable materials like

stainless steel, cast iron, or ceramic, as they have a longer lifespan and can be recycled at the end of their usefulness.

- Reusable food storage containers: Reduce the use of disposable plastic bags and food wraps by using reusable food storage containers. Opt for glass, stainless steel, or BPA-free plastic containers that are microwave-safe and easy to clean.
- Compost bin: Set up a compost bin in your kitchen to collect food scraps and other organic waste. Composting helps divert waste from landfills and produces nutrient-rich soil for gardening.
- Reusable kitchen essentials: Replace disposable items with reusable alternatives. Use cloth towels instead of paper towels, fabric napkins instead of paper ones, and reusable silicone or beeswax wraps instead of plastic wraps.
- Water-saving devices: Install aerators on faucets and a low-flow showerhead to reduce water consumption in the kitchen. Collect and reuse water from rinsing fruits and vegetables or cooking to water plants.
- Recycling and waste management systems: Set up a convenient recycling station in your kitchen with separate bins for paper, plastic, glass, and metal. Consider composting systems for food waste and use recycling and waste management services provided by your local municipality.

By equipping your kitchen with sustainable tools and equipment, you can minimize energy and water consumption, reduce waste, and create an environmentally friendly cooking space.

## Minimizing waste and utilizing leftovers

Minimizing waste and utilizing leftovers are important practices that contribute to sustainability and help reduce the environmental impact of our food consumption. By making the most of the food we have and reducing food waste, we can save resources, reduce greenhouse gas emissions, and save money. Here are some strategies for minimizing waste and utilizing leftovers:

- Plan meals and make a shopping list: Before grocery shopping, plan your meals for the week and make a shopping list. This helps you buy only what you need, reducing the chances of food going to waste.
- Proper storage: Store perishable foods properly to extend their shelf life. Use airtight containers or beeswax wraps to keep fruits, vegetables, and leftovers fresh. Label and date containers to ensure you use the oldest items first.
- First in, first out: When organizing your fridge and pantry, practice the "first in, first out" principle. Place newly purchased items at the back and bring older items to the front. This ensures that items with a shorter shelf life are used before they spoil.
- Portion control: Prepare and serve appropriate

portions to avoid leftovers that may go to waste. Start with smaller portions and allow people to serve themselves seconds if desired.

- Get creative with leftovers: Transform leftovers into new meals by repurposing them. For example, leftover roasted chicken can be used in sandwiches, soups, or salads. Vegetable scraps can be used to make broth or added to stir-fries. Be creative and experiment with different recipes to make the most of your leftovers.
- Freeze leftovers: If you can't consume leftovers immediately, freeze them in individual or family-sized portions. Properly label and date the containers for easy identification. Frozen leftovers can be used for quick meals on busy days.
- Donate excess food: If you have excess food that you won't be able to consume, consider donating it to local food banks, shelters, or community organizations. This helps reduce food waste while supporting those in need.
- Compost food scraps: Set up a compost bin or participate in community composting programs to divert food scraps from landfills. Composting turns organic waste into nutrient-rich soil, which can be used in gardens or donated to local farmers.

By minimizing waste and utilizing leftovers, we can make a significant impact on reducing food waste and its environmental consequences.

**Meal planning and prepping for efficient and eco-friendly**

## cooking

Meal planning and prepping are effective strategies for efficient and eco-friendly cooking. By dedicating some time to plan and prepare meals in advance, you can reduce food waste, save energy, and make healthier food choices. Here are some tips for meal planning and prepping:

- Plan your meals: Set aside a specific time each week to plan your meals. Consider your schedule, dietary preferences, and the ingredients you already have. Plan a variety of meals that incorporate seasonal produce and use similar ingredients to minimize waste.
- Make a shopping list: Based on your meal plan, create a shopping list. Stick to the list to avoid impulse purchases and unnecessary food waste.
- Cook in batches: Prepare larger quantities of meals and cook in batches. This saves time and energy since you're utilizing the oven or stove less frequently. Portion the cooked food into individual containers for easy grab-and-go meals throughout the week.
- Use leftovers creatively: Incorporate planned leftovers into your meal plan. For example, roast a whole chicken one night and use the leftovers for sandwiches, salads, or stir-fries later in the week. Be creative and find ways to repurpose ingredients to minimize waste.
- Prep ingredients in advance: Wash, chop, and prep ingredients in advance to save time during

the week. Store prepped ingredients in airtight containers or reusable bags in the fridge, ready to be used in recipes.

- Optimize kitchen appliances: Use kitchen appliances efficiently to save energy. For example, when using the oven, cook multiple dishes at once to maximize its capacity. Use slow cookers or pressure cookers to save time and energy when preparing meals.
- Store food properly: Proper storage extends the shelf life of ingredients and prepared meals. Use airtight containers or freezer-safe bags to store leftovers, prepped ingredients, and batch-cooked meals. Label and date containers to keep track of freshness.
- Embrace seasonal and local produce: Plan meals around seasonal and local produce. Not only does this support local farmers, but it also reduces the environmental impact of long-distance transportation.
- Consider reusable meal containers: Invest in reusable meal containers made from eco-friendly materials. These containers eliminate the need for single-use plastic containers or wraps.
- Monitor and adjust: Pay attention to the success of your meal planning and prepping efforts. Adjust your plan based on your family's preferences and the amount of food that goes to waste. Continually refine your approach to minimize waste and improve efficiency.

By incorporating meal planning and prepping into your routine, you can save time, reduce food waste, and make cooking a more enjoyable and sustainable experience.

## Navigating Eating Out and Social Situations

**Tips for making sustainable choices at restaurants**

Making sustainable choices when dining out is an important part of adopting a lean and green lifestyle. Here are some tips to help you make sustainable choices at restaurants:

- Choose local and seasonal options: Look for restaurants that prioritize locally sourced ingredients and offer seasonal menus. Locally sourced food reduces the carbon footprint associated with transportation, supports local farmers, and promotes fresher and more flavorful meals.
- Opt for plant-based options: Choosing plant-based dishes can have a significant positive impact on the environment. Plant-based meals require fewer resources to produce and reduce greenhouse gas emissions. Look for vegetarian or vegan options on the menu or request modifications to existing dishes.
- Minimize food waste: Be mindful of portion sizes and consider sharing meals with others. If you have leftovers, ask for a take-out container to avoid food waste. Some restaurants have initiatives to reduce food waste, so inquire about their policies or partnerships with local food

banks.

- Choose sustainably sourced seafood: If you enjoy seafood, opt for sustainably sourced options. Look for restaurants that follow sustainable seafood practices and support organizations such as MSC (Marine Stewardship Council) or ASC (Aquaculture Stewardship Council).
- Bring your own reusable containers: If you know you'll have leftovers, come prepared with your own reusable containers to avoid using disposable ones. This helps reduce single-use plastic waste and promotes sustainable practices.
- Skip the plastic straws and utensils: Request drinks without plastic straws or bring your own reusable straw. If possible, choose restaurants that use reusable or compostable utensils instead of single-use plastic ones.
- Support environmentally conscious restaurants: Research and support restaurants that prioritize sustainability and eco-friendly practices. Look for certifications such as LEED (Leadership in Energy and Environmental Design) or Green Restaurant Association (GRA) certifications.

## Green alternatives when dining out

When dining out, there are several green alternatives you can choose to reduce your environmental impact. Here are some ideas for making greener choices when dining out:

- Opt for tap water: Choose tap water instead of bottled water to reduce plastic waste. If you prefer filtered water, bring your own reusable water bottle.

- Bring your own reusable containers and bags: When ordering takeout or getting leftovers, bring your own reusable containers and bags. This helps reduce the use of single-use packaging and supports sustainable practices.
- Choose restaurants that prioritize local and organic ingredients: Look for restaurants that prioritize sourcing local and organic ingredients. These establishments support local farmers, reduce transportation emissions, and often offer healthier and more sustainable food options.
- Support restaurants with eco-friendly practices: Seek out restaurants that implement eco-friendly practices such as using energy-efficient appliances, recycling and composting, and minimizing waste. These establishments contribute to a more sustainable food industry.
- Look for vegetarian and vegan options: Even if you're not vegetarian or vegan, choosing plant-based options when dining out can significantly reduce your carbon footprint. Many restaurants now offer delicious and creative plant-based dishes that are both satisfying and sustainable.
- Choose sustainable seafood: If you enjoy seafood, opt for sustainably sourced options. Look for restaurants that follow sustainable seafood practices and offer certified sustainable seafood choices.
- Consider the distance traveled: When choosing a restaurant, consider the distance you need to travel. Opting for a restaurant closer to home

reduces carbon emissions from transportation.

## Hosting eco-friendly gatherings and parties

Hosting eco-friendly gatherings and parties allows you to enjoy celebrations while minimizing the environmental impact. Here are some ideas for hosting eco-friendly gatherings:

- Send digital invitations: Instead of traditional paper invitations, send digital invitations or use online platforms for event planning. This reduces paper waste and makes it easier for guests to RSVP.
- Use sustainable decorations: Opt for reusable and eco-friendly decorations such as biodegradable balloons, paper or fabric banners, potted plants, or flowers from local and sustainable sources. Avoid single-use plastic decorations.
- Choose sustainable tableware: Use reusable plates, cups, and utensils instead of disposable ones. If using disposable tableware is necessary, opt for compostable or biodegradable options made from materials like bamboo or sugarcane.
- Serve locally sourced and seasonal food: Choose locally sourced and seasonal ingredients for your menu. Supporting local farmers reduces the carbon footprint associated with transportation, and seasonal produce often tastes better.
- Minimize food waste: Plan your menu carefully to avoid excess food. Encourage guests to bring reusable containers to take home leftovers, or

consider donating excess food to local food banks or shelters.
- Provide recycling and composting bins: Make it easy for guests to recycle by setting up clearly labeled recycling bins. If possible, provide a compost bin for food scraps and compostable items.

## Conclusion: Embracing a Lean and Green Lifestyle

### Recap of the key principles and benefits of lean and green eating

Lean and green eating combines the principles of both healthy and sustainable food choices. Here is a recap of the key principles and benefits of lean and green eating:

Principles of Lean and Green Eating:

- Focus on whole, unprocessed foods: Choose foods in their most natural state, such as fruits, vegetables, whole grains, legumes, and lean proteins. These foods are nutrient-dense and provide a range of vitamins, minerals, and antioxidants.
- Minimize processed and packaged foods: Processed foods often contain added sugars, unhealthy fats, and artificial ingredients. By reducing their consumption, you can improve your overall health and reduce your

environmental impact.

- Prioritize plant-based meals: Incorporate more plant-based meals into your diet by choosing fruits, vegetables, legumes, nuts, and seeds. Plant-based meals are generally lower in environmental impact and can provide numerous health benefits.
- Choose sustainably sourced proteins: When consuming animal-based proteins, opt for options that are sustainably and ethically sourced. Look for certifications such as organic, grass-fed, or free-range to ensure responsible farming practices.

Benefits of Lean and Green Eating:

- Improved health and weight management: Lean and green eating focuses on nutrient-dense foods, which can support overall health and weight management. A diet rich in fruits, vegetables, whole grains, and lean proteins can help reduce the risk of chronic diseases and maintain a healthy weight.
- Environmental sustainability: By choosing sustainable and locally sourced foods, you can reduce your carbon footprint and support a more environmentally friendly food system. Eating lower on the food chain, such as incorporating more plant-based meals, helps conserve resources and reduces greenhouse gas emissions.
- Enhanced energy and vitality: The nutrients found in whole, unprocessed foods can provide sustained energy throughout the day. Lean and green eating promotes stable blood sugar levels and reduces the consumption of foods that may

cause energy crashes.

- Support for local farmers and communities: Prioritizing locally sourced and seasonal foods helps support local farmers and communities. It strengthens the local economy and reduces the dependence on long-distance transportation, thereby reducing carbon emissions.

## Sustainable habits for long-term success

Adopting sustainable habits is crucial for long-term success in maintaining a lean and green lifestyle. Here are some sustainable habits to incorporate into your daily routine:

- Meal planning and prepping: Plan your meals in advance to minimize food waste and make healthier choices. Set aside time each week to prepare and portion meals, ensuring you have nutritious options readily available.
- Choose reusable alternatives: Reduce single-use plastics by opting for reusable alternatives. Bring your own shopping bags, water bottles, coffee mugs, and utensils when you're on the go.
- Reduce food waste: Practice mindful grocery shopping, proper food storage, and creative ways to utilize leftovers. Minimizing food waste not only benefits the environment but also saves money.
- Support local and sustainable agriculture: Seek out local farmers' markets or join community-

supported agriculture (CSA) programs to support local and sustainable food sources. This helps reduce the environmental impact of long-distance transportation and supports local economies.

- Conserve water and energy: Incorporate habits such as turning off lights when not in use, using energy-efficient appliances, and conserving water by fixing leaks and using water-saving fixtures.
- Reduce reliance on animal products: Incorporate more plant-based meals into your diet. Choose alternatives to animal-based products, such as plant-based proteins, and explore a variety of plant-based recipes.
- Compost food scraps: Start a composting system at home to reduce organic waste and create nutrient-rich soil for your garden. Composting diverts waste from landfills and reduces greenhouse gas emissions.
- Engage in conscious consumerism: Consider the environmental impact of the products you purchase. Choose sustainable and ethically produced goods, support companies with transparent and eco-friendly practices, and reduce unnecessary consumption.

**Inspiring readers to make a positive impact on their health and the environment**

Making a positive impact on both personal health and the environment is an empowering journey. Here are some ways to inspire readers to embrace a lean and green lifestyle:

- Education and awareness: Share information about the benefits of lean and green eating, sustainable practices, and their impact on personal health and the environment. Empower readers with knowledge to make informed choices.
- Highlight success stories: Share stories of individuals or communities who have successfully embraced a lean and green lifestyle. These stories can inspire and motivate readers to take action and make positive changes in their own lives.
- Provide practical tips and guidance: Offer practical tips, step-by-step guides, and recipes to help readers transition to a lean and green lifestyle. Make it accessible and show how small changes can make a significant impact.
- Emphasize the interconnectedness: Help readers understand how their personal choices and actions can contribute to a larger movement toward sustainability. Highlight the collective impact of individuals working together for a healthier planet.
- Foster a supportive community: Create a platform or community where readers can connect, share experiences, and provide support to one another. Encourage dialogue, questions, and the exchange of ideas to foster a sense of belonging and motivation.
- Showcase the variety and deliciousness: Highlight the wide range of delicious and satisfying

lean and green recipes. Show that healthy and sustainable eating doesn't mean sacrificing taste or enjoyment.

- Celebrate progress, not perfection: Encourage readers to embrace progress rather than striving for perfection. Recognize that small changes and consistent efforts can lead to significant and lasting impact.

By inspiring readers to make a positive impact on their health and the environment, you can motivate them to embrace a lean and green lifestyle that benefits not only themselves but also the planet we all call home.

# CHAPTER TWO

## Energizing Smoothie Bowls and Plant-Based Breakfasts

**Description:**

Start your day off right with these energizing smoothie bowls and plant-based breakfasts. Packed with vitamins, minerals, and antioxidants, these nutritious meals will provide a delicious and refreshing start to your morning. Whether you prefer fruity flavors or rich and creamy textures, there's a recipe here to satisfy every taste bud.

**Ingredients:**

- 1 ripe banana
- 1 cup frozen berries (such as strawberries, blueberries, or raspberries)
- 1/2 cup almond milk
- 2 tablespoons chia seeds
- 1 tablespoon almond butter
- 1 tablespoon honey or maple syrup
- Toppings of your choice: sliced fruits, granola, shredded coconut, nuts, and seeds

**Instructions:**

- In a blender, combine the ripe banana, frozen berries, almond milk, chia seeds, almond butter, and honey or maple syrup.
- Blend until smooth and creamy, adding more almond milk if needed to achieve the desired consistency.
- Pour the smoothie into a bowl and top with your favorite toppings, such as sliced fruits, granola, shredded coconut, nuts, and seeds.
- Enjoy immediately and feel the energizing power of this delicious plant-based breakfast!

**Nutritional Information:**

Calories: 350

Protein: 8g

Fat: 12g

Carbohydrates: 55g

Fiber: 10g

# High-Fiber Whole Grain Cereals and Muesli Options

**Description:**

Get your daily dose of fiber with these high-fiber whole grain cereals and muesli options. These breakfast recipes are not only delicious but also packed with essential nutrients to keep you feeling full and satisfied throughout the day. From crunchy granola clusters to hearty oatmeal, these recipes will make your mornings extra wholesome.

**Ingredients**:

- 1 cup rolled oats
- 1/4 cup chopped nuts (such as almonds, walnuts, or pecans)
- 2 tablespoons chia seeds
- 2 tablespoons ground flaxseed
- 1 tablespoon honey or maple syrup
- 1 cup plant-based milk (such as almond milk or oat milk)
- Fresh fruits and yogurt for topping (optional)

**Instructions**:

- In a mixing bowl, combine the rolled oats, chopped nuts, chia seeds, ground flaxseed, honey or maple syrup, and plant-based milk.
- Stir well to ensure all the ingredients are evenly mixed.
- Cover the bowl and refrigerate overnight or for at least 4 hours to allow the mixture to thicken.
- In the morning, give the cereal a good stir and top with fresh fruits and a dollop of yogurt if desired.
- Enjoy the wholesome goodness of this high-fiber breakfast that will keep you fueled for the day ahead!

**Nutritional Information**:

Calories: 300

Protein: 10g

Fat: 15g

Carbohydrates: 35g

Fiber: 12g

## Sustainable Protein-Packed Breakfast Options

**Description:**

Start your day with sustainable protein-packed breakfast options that are not only good for you but also good for the planet. These recipes feature plant-based proteins that are rich in nutrients and environmentally friendly. From tofu scrambles to chickpea omelets, these delicious breakfast ideas will keep you satisfied and support your sustainable lifestyle.

**Ingredients:**

- 1 block of firm tofu
- 1 tablespoon nutritional yeast
- 1/2 teaspoon turmeric
- 1/2 teaspoon garlic powder
- 1/2 teaspoon onion powder
- Salt and pepper to taste

- 2 tablespoons olive oil
- Assorted vegetables (such as spinach, bell peppers, mushrooms, and onions)

**Instructions**:

- Drain the tofu and press it with a paper towel to remove excess moisture.
- Crumble the tofu into a bowl and add nutritional yeast, turmeric, garlic powder, onion powder, salt, and pepper.
- Mix well to evenly coat the tofu with the seasoning.
- Heat olive oil in a skillet over medium heat and add the seasoned tofu.
- Cook for 5-7 minutes, stirring occasionally, until the tofu is golden and slightly crispy.
- Add the assorted vegetables to the skillet and cook for an additional 3-4 minutes, until the vegetables are tender.
- Serve the protein-packed scramble on toast or alongside whole grain bread, and enjoy a sustainable breakfast that's both delicious and good for the planet!

**Nutritional Information:**

Calories: 250

Protein: 15g

Fat: 12g

Carbohydrates: 20g

Fiber: 5g

# Creative Ideas for Incorporating Vegetables into Breakfast

**Description**:

Get your daily dose of vegetables with these creative ideas for incorporating them into breakfast. Who said veggies were just for lunch and dinner? These recipes prove that vegetables can add a burst of flavor and nutrition to your morning meals. From zucchini pancakes to sweet potato toast, these breakfast ideas will make you fall in love with veggies all over again.

**Ingredients**:

- 1 medium zucchini, grated
- 1/4 cup whole wheat flour
- 1/4 cup grated Parmesan cheese
- 1/4 teaspoon baking powder
- 1/4 teaspoon salt
- 1/4 teaspoon black pepper
- 2 eggs
- Olive oil for cooking

**Instructions**:

- In a mixing bowl, combine the grated zucchini,

whole wheat flour, Parmesan cheese, baking powder, salt, black pepper, and eggs.
- Mix well until all the ingredients are thoroughly combined.
- Heat a drizzle of olive oil in a non-stick skillet over medium heat.
- Spoon the zucchini batter onto the skillet, forming small pancakes.
- Cook for 2-3 minutes on each side, until golden brown and cooked through.
- Serve the zucchini pancakes with a side of fresh salad or yogurt, and savor the deliciousness of vegetables in your breakfast!

**Nutritional Information:**

Calories: 180

Protein: 10g

Fat: 8g

Carbohydrates: 15g

Fiber: 4g

# Nutrient-Dense Salad Combinations

**Description:**

Elevate your salad game with these nutrient-dense salad combinations. Packed with vitamins, minerals, and fiber, these salads will not only tantalize your taste buds but also nourish your body. From vibrant greens to colorful vegetables, these salad recipes are a delicious way to incorporate more nutrients into your daily meals.

**Ingredients**:

- 4 cups mixed salad greens
- 1 cup cherry tomatoes, halved
- 1 cucumber, sliced
- 1 bell pepper, diced
- ½ red onion, thinly sliced
- ¼ cup sliced almonds
- ¼ cup crumbled feta cheese
- 2 tablespoons extra virgin olive oil
- 1 tablespoon balsamic vinegar
- Salt and pepper to taste

**Instructions**:

- In a large salad bowl, combine the mixed salad greens, cherry tomatoes, cucumber, bell pepper, red onion, sliced almonds, and crumbled feta cheese.
- In a small bowl, whisk together the extra virgin olive oil, balsamic vinegar, salt, and pepper to make the dressing.
- Drizzle the dressing over the salad and toss gently to coat all the ingredients.
- Serve immediately and enjoy the burst of flavors and nutrients in this nutrient-dense salad combination.

**Nutritional Information:**

Calories: 180

Protein: 6g

Fat: 14g

Carbohydrates: 10g

Fiber: 4g

## Homemade Dressings and Vinaigrettes

**Description:**

Enhance the flavors of your salads with these homemade dressings and vinaigrettes. Say goodbye to store-bought dressings filled with preservatives and additives, and say hello to fresh and flavorful dressings made with simple ingredients. These recipes will take your salads to the next level and impress your taste buds.

**Ingredients:**

Lemon Vinaigrette:

- Juice of 1 lemon
- 2 tablespoons extra virgin olive oil
- 1 teaspoon Dijon mustard

- 1 garlic clove, minced
- Salt and pepper to taste

Honey Mustard Dressing:

- 2 tablespoons Dijon mustard
- 1 tablespoon honey
- 2 tablespoons apple cider vinegar
- 3 tablespoons extra virgin olive oil
- Salt and pepper to taste

## Instructions:

Lemon Vinaigrette:

- In a small bowl, whisk together the lemon juice, extra virgin olive oil, Dijon mustard, minced garlic, salt, and pepper.
- Adjust the seasoning according to your taste preferences.
- Drizzle the lemon vinaigrette over your favorite salad and toss to coat.

Honey Mustard Dressing:

- In a small bowl, whisk together the Dijon mustard, honey, apple cider vinegar, extra virgin olive oil, salt, and pepper.
- Taste and adjust the sweetness or tanginess by adding more honey or vinegar, if desired.
- Drizzle the honey mustard dressing over your salad and enjoy the homemade goodness.
- Nutritional Information:
- The nutritional information for the dressings may vary based on the specific ingredients

used. Please refer to the individual ingredients' nutritional labels for accurate information.

## Innovative Vegetable-Based Side Dishes

**Description**:

Add a twist to your side dishes with these innovative vegetable-based recipes. From roasted cauliflower steaks to zucchini noodles, these dishes are not only creative but also packed with vitamins and minerals. Elevate your meals with these delicious and nutritious vegetable side dishes.

**Ingredients**:

Roasted Cauliflower Steaks:

- 1 large head of cauliflower
- 2 tablespoons olive oil
- 1 teaspoon garlic powder
- ½ teaspoon paprika
- Salt and pepper to taste

Zucchini Noodles with Pesto:

- 2-3 zucchinis
- ¼ cup homemade or store-bought pesto
- Cherry tomatoes, halved (optional)
- Fresh basil leaves for garnish (optional)

**Instructions**:

Roasted Cauliflower Steaks:

- Preheat the oven to 425°F (220°C).
- Slice the cauliflower into 1-inch thick steaks, keeping the stem intact.
- Place the cauliflower steaks on a baking sheet lined with parchment paper.
- In a small bowl, mix together the olive oil, garlic powder, paprika, salt, and pepper.
- Brush both sides of the cauliflower steaks with the oil mixture.
- Roast in the oven for 20-25 minutes, flipping halfway through, until golden and tender.

Zucchini Noodles with Pesto:

- Use a spiralizer or vegetable peeler to create zucchini noodles.
- In a large pan, heat a drizzle of olive oil over medium heat.
- Add the zucchini noodles and cook for 2-3 minutes, until slightly softened.
- Remove from heat and toss the zucchini noodles with the pesto sauce.
- If desired, add cherry tomatoes for extra freshness and garnish with fresh basil leaves.
- Serve as a flavorful vegetable-based side dish and enjoy the creativity on your plate.

**Nutritional Information:**

The nutritional information for the vegetable-based side dishes may vary based on the specific ingredients used.

Please refer to the individual ingredients' nutritional labels for accurate information.

## Sustainable Grain and Legume Salads

**Description:**

Enjoy the goodness of sustainable ingredients with these grain and legume salads. Packed with protein, fiber, and a variety of nutrients, these salads are not only satisfying but also environmentally friendly. From quinoa and black bean salads to lentil and couscous combinations, these recipes will nourish your body and support sustainable eating.

**Ingredients:**

Quinoa and Black Bean Salad:

- 1 cup cooked quinoa
- 1 can black beans, rinsed and drained
- 1 bell pepper, diced
- ½ red onion, finely chopped
- ¼ cup chopped fresh cilantro
- Juice of 1 lime
- 2 tablespoons extra virgin olive oil
- Salt and pepper to taste

Lentil and Couscous Salad:

- 1 cup cooked lentils

- 1 cup cooked couscous
- 1 cucumber, diced
- 1 tomato, diced
- ¼ cup chopped fresh parsley
- 2 tablespoons lemon juice
- 2 tablespoons extra virgin olive oil
- Salt and pepper to taste

**Instructions**:

Quinoa and Black Bean Salad:

- In a large bowl, combine the cooked quinoa, black beans, diced bell pepper, finely chopped red onion, and chopped fresh cilantro.
- In a separate small bowl, whisk together the lime juice, extra virgin olive oil, salt, and pepper.
- Pour the dressing over the salad ingredients and toss to combine.
- Adjust the seasoning according to your taste preferences.
- Let the flavors meld together for at least 15 minutes before serving.

Lentil and Couscous Salad:

- In a large bowl, combine the cooked lentils, cooked couscous, diced cucumber, diced tomato, and chopped fresh parsley.
- In a separate small bowl, whisk together the lemon juice, extra virgin olive oil, salt, and pepper.
- Drizzle the dressing over the salad ingredients and toss gently to coat.
- Taste and adjust the seasoning as needed.
- Allow the salad to sit for a short while to let the

flavors mingle before serving.

**Nutritional Information:**

The nutritional information for the grain and legume salads may vary based on the specific ingredients used. Please refer to the individual ingredients' nutritional labels for accurate information.

## Hearty Vegetable Soups and Broth-Based Stews

**Description**:

Warm your soul with these hearty vegetable soups and broth-based stews. Packed with a medley of nutritious vegetables and aromatic herbs, these comforting recipes are perfect for chilly days or whenever you crave a nourishing bowl of goodness. From chunky minestrone to creamy butternut squash soup, these dishes will keep you satisfied and satisfied.

**Ingredients**:

Chunky Minestrone:

- 1 tablespoon olive oil
- 1 onion, diced
- 2 cloves of garlic, minced
- 2 carrots, diced

- 2 celery stalks, diced
- 1 zucchini, diced
- 1 cup diced tomatoes
- 4 cups vegetable broth
- 1 cup cooked kidney beans
- 1 cup cooked small pasta (such as elbow or shell pasta)
- 1 teaspoon dried oregano
- 1 teaspoon dried basil
- Salt and pepper to taste
- Fresh parsley for garnish (optional)

Creamy Butternut Squash Soup:

- 1 medium butternut squash, peeled, seeded, and cubed
- 1 onion, chopped
- 2 cloves of garlic, minced
- 4 cups vegetable broth
- ½ cup coconut milk
- 1 teaspoon ground cumin
- ½ teaspoon ground cinnamon
- Salt and pepper to taste
- Toasted pumpkin seeds for garnish (optional)

**Instructions**:

Chunky Minestrone:

- Heat olive oil in a large pot over medium heat.
- Add diced onion, minced garlic, diced carrots, diced celery, and diced zucchini. Sauté for 5 minutes until the vegetables start to soften.
- Stir in diced tomatoes and vegetable broth. Bring to a boil.

- Reduce heat to low, cover, and simmer for 20-25 minutes.
- Add cooked kidney beans and cooked pasta to the pot. Season with dried oregano, dried basil, salt, and pepper. Simmer for an additional 5 minutes.
- Serve the chunky minestrone soup hot, garnished with fresh parsley if desired.

Creamy Butternut Squash Soup:

- In a large pot, combine butternut squash, chopped onion, minced garlic, and vegetable broth. Bring to a boil.
- Reduce heat to low, cover, and simmer for 20-25 minutes or until the butternut squash is tender.
- Using an immersion blender or regular blender, blend the soup until smooth and creamy.
- Stir in coconut milk, ground cumin, ground cinnamon, salt, and pepper. Simmer for an additional 5 minutes.
- Serve the creamy butternut squash soup hot, garnished with toasted pumpkin seeds if desired.

**Nutritional Information:**

The nutritional information for the vegetable soups and stews may vary based on the specific ingredients used. Please refer to the individual ingredients' nutritional labels for accurate information.

# Plant-Based Protein Soups and Chilies

**Description**:

Get your protein fix with these plant-based protein soups and chilies. Packed with legumes, tofu, and hearty vegetables, these recipes are not only satisfying but also rich in nutrients. From lentil soup to vegan chili, these plant-based options will keep you warm and fueled throughout the day.

**Ingredients**:

Lentil Soup:

- 1 cup dried green or brown lentils
- 1 onion, diced
- 2 carrots, diced
- 2 celery stalks, diced
- 3 cloves of garlic, minced
- 4 cups vegetable broth
- 1 bay leaf
- 1 teaspoon ground cumin
- ½ teaspoon ground coriander
- ¼ teaspoon red pepper flakes (optional)
- Salt and pepper to taste
- Fresh parsley for garnish (optional)

Vegan Chili:

- 1 tablespoon olive oil
- 1 onion, diced
- 2 cloves of garlic, minced
- 1 bell pepper, diced

- 1 zucchini, diced
- 1 can diced tomatoes
- 1 can kidney beans, rinsed and drained
- 1 can black beans, rinsed and drained
- 1 cup vegetable broth
- 1 tablespoon chili powder
- 1 teaspoon ground cumin
- ½ teaspoon paprika
- Salt and pepper to taste
- Fresh cilantro for garnish (optional)

**Instructions**:

Lentil Soup:

- Rinse the lentils under cold water and set aside.
- In a large pot, heat olive oil over medium heat. Add diced onion, diced carrots, diced celery, and minced garlic. Sauté for 5 minutes until the vegetables start to soften.
- Add lentils, vegetable broth, bay leaf, ground cumin, ground coriander, red pepper flakes (if using), salt, and pepper. Bring to a boil.
- Reduce heat to low, cover, and simmer for 25-30 minutes or until the lentils are tender.
- Remove the bay leaf and adjust the seasoning if needed.
- Serve the lentil soup hot, garnished with fresh parsley if desired.

Vegan Chili:

- Heat olive oil in a large pot over medium heat. Add diced onion, minced garlic, diced bell pepper, and diced zucchini. Sauté for 5 minutes until the

vegetables start to soften.
- Stir in diced tomatoes, kidney beans, black beans, vegetable broth, chili powder, ground cumin, paprika, salt, and pepper. Bring to a boil.
- Reduce heat to low, cover, and simmer for 20-25 minutes to allow the flavors to meld together.
- Adjust the seasoning if needed.
- Serve the vegan chili hot, garnished with fresh cilantro if desired.

**Nutritional Information:**

The nutritional information for the plant-based protein soups and chilies may vary based on the specific ingredients used. Please refer to the individual ingredients' nutritional labels for accurate information.

## Sustainable Seafood and Fish-Based Soups

**Description**:

Indulge in the flavors of the sea with these sustainable seafood and fish-based soups. Packed with oceanic goodness and aromatic herbs, these recipes showcase the natural flavors of seafood while promoting sustainable choices. From classic fish chowder to spicy shrimp soup, these soups will transport you to coastal destinations and leave you craving more.

**Ingredients**:

Classic Fish Chowder:

- 1 tablespoon butter or olive oil
- 1 onion, diced
- 2 carrots, diced
- 2 celery stalks, diced
- 2 cloves of garlic, minced
- 4 cups fish or vegetable broth
- 2 cups diced potatoes
- 1 bay leaf
- ½ teaspoon dried thyme
- 1 cup milk or coconut milk
- 1 pound white fish fillets (such as cod or haddock), cut into bite-sized pieces
- Salt and pepper to taste
- Fresh parsley for garnish (optional)

Spicy Shrimp Soup:

- 1 tablespoon olive oil
- 1 onion, diced
- 2 cloves of garlic, minced
- 1 bell pepper, diced
- 1 jalapeno pepper, seeded and minced
- 4 cups seafood or vegetable broth
- 1 can diced tomatoes
- 1 teaspoon smoked paprika
- ½ teaspoon ground cumin
- ¼ teaspoon cayenne pepper (adjust to taste)
- 1 pound shrimp, peeled and deveined
- Juice of 1 lime
- Salt and pepper to taste

- Fresh cilantro for garnish (optional)

**Instructions**:

Classic Fish Chowder:

- In a large pot, melt butter or heat olive oil over medium heat. Add diced onion, diced carrots, diced celery, and minced garlic. Sauté for 5 minutes until the vegetables start to soften.
- Add fish or vegetable broth, diced potatoes, bay leaf, and dried thyme. Bring to a boil.
- Reduce heat to low, cover, and simmer for 15-20 minutes or until the potatoes are tender.
- Stir in milk or coconut milk and add the fish fillets. Cook for an additional 5 minutes or until the fish is cooked through.
- Season with salt and pepper.
- Serve the classic fish chowder hot, garnished with fresh parsley if desired.

Spicy Shrimp Soup:

- Heat olive oil in a large pot over medium heat. Add diced onion, minced garlic, diced bell pepper, and minced jalapeno pepper. Sauté for 5 minutes until the vegetables start to soften.
- Stir in seafood or vegetable broth, diced tomatoes, smoked paprika, ground cumin, and cayenne pepper. Bring to a boil.
- Reduce heat to low, cover, and simmer for 15 minutes to allow the flavors to meld together.
- Add shrimp and cook for an additional 3-5 minutes or until the shrimp are pink and cooked through.

- Stir in lime juice and season with salt and pepper.
- Serve the spicy shrimp soup hot, garnished with fresh cilantro if desired.

**Nutritional Information:**

The nutritional information for the seafood and fish-based soups may vary based on the specific ingredients used. Please refer to the individual ingredients' nutritional labels for accurate information.

## Flavorful Plant-Based Entrées

**Description:**

Indulge in these flavorful plant-based entrées that showcase the versatility of plant-based ingredients. From hearty grain bowls to creative vegetable-based dishes, these recipes are packed with vibrant flavors and nutrients. Whether you follow a vegetarian or vegan lifestyle or simply enjoy incorporating more plant-based meals into your diet, these entrées will satisfy your cravings and delight your taste buds.

**Ingredients:**

Quinoa and Roasted Vegetable Bowl:

- 1 cup cooked quinoa
- Assorted roasted vegetables (e.g., bell peppers, zucchini, eggplant, mushrooms)
- 2 cups mixed greens
- ¼ cup crumbled feta cheese (optional)
- Lemon tahini dressing:
- 2 tablespoons tahini
- Juice of 1 lemon
- 1 tablespoon extra virgin olive oil
- Salt and pepper to taste

Cauliflower Curry with Chickpeas:

- 1 small head of cauliflower, cut into florets
- 1 can chickpeas, rinsed and drained
- 1 onion, diced
- 2 cloves of garlic, minced
- 1 tablespoon curry powder
- 1 teaspoon ground cumin
- 1 teaspoon ground turmeric
- 1 can coconut milk
- 1 cup vegetable broth
- Fresh cilantro for garnish (optional)
- Cooked rice or naan bread for serving

**Instructions**:

Quinoa and Roasted Vegetable Bowl:

- Preheat the oven to 425°F (220°C).
- Toss the assorted vegetables with olive oil, salt, and pepper on a baking sheet. Roast for 20-25 minutes until tender and slightly charred.
- In a bowl, assemble the cooked quinoa, roasted vegetables, mixed greens, and crumbled feta

cheese (if using).
- In a small bowl, whisk together tahini, lemon juice, extra virgin olive oil, salt, and pepper to make the dressing.
- Drizzle the lemon tahini dressing over the quinoa and roasted vegetable bowl.
- Toss gently to combine all the ingredients.
- Serve the flavorful plant-based entrée bowl and enjoy the burst of flavors.

Cauliflower Curry with Chickpeas:

- In a large pot, heat olive oil over medium heat. Add diced onion and minced garlic. Sauté for 5 minutes until the onion becomes translucent.
- Add cauliflower florets, chickpeas, curry powder, ground cumin, and ground turmeric. Stir well to coat the cauliflower and chickpeas with the spices.
- Pour in the coconut milk and vegetable broth. Bring to a boil.
- Reduce heat to low, cover, and simmer for 15-20 minutes or until the cauliflower is tender.
- Garnish with fresh cilantro if desired.
- Serve the cauliflower curry with chickpeas over cooked rice or with naan bread for a satisfying plant-based entrée.

**Nutritional Information:**

The nutritional information for the plant-based entrées may vary based on the specific ingredients used. Please refer to the individual ingredients' nutritional labels for accurate information.

# Sustainable Seafood and Fish Recipes

**Description:**

Dive into the world of sustainable seafood and fish with these delicious and nutritious recipes. From seared salmon to grilled shrimp, these dishes highlight the natural flavors of seafood while promoting sustainable fishing practices. Enjoy the omega-3 fatty acids and essential nutrients that seafood provides while supporting the health of our oceans.

**Ingredients:**

Seared Sesame Tuna:

- 2 tuna steaks
- 2 tablespoons soy sauce or tamari sauce
- 1 tablespoon sesame oil
- 1 tablespoon rice vinegar
- 1 tablespoon honey or maple syrup
- 1 tablespoon sesame seeds
- Sliced green onions for garnish (optional)

Grilled Lemon Herb Shrimp:

- 1 pound shrimp, peeled and deveined
- Juice and zest of 1 lemon
- 2 tablespoons olive oil
- 2 cloves of garlic, minced

- 1 tablespoon chopped fresh parsley
- 1 tablespoon chopped fresh dill
- Salt and pepper to taste
- Skewers for grilling (if using wooden skewers, soak them in water for 30 minutes before grilling)

**Instructions**:

Seared Sesame Tuna:

- In a shallow dish, whisk together soy sauce, sesame oil, rice vinegar, and honey or maple syrup to make the marinade.
- Place the tuna steaks in the marinade and let them marinate for 15-30 minutes, flipping them halfway through.
- Heat a skillet or grill pan over high heat.
- Remove the tuna steaks from the marinade, allowing any excess marinade to drip off.
- Sprinkle sesame seeds on a plate and press the tuna steaks into the seeds, coating both sides.
- Sear the tuna steaks for 1-2 minutes on each side for rare to medium-rare doneness, or cook to your preferred level of doneness.
- Remove the tuna steaks from the heat and let them rest for a few minutes before slicing.
- Garnish with sliced green onions if desired.
- Serve the seared sesame tuna as a main dish or slice it for use in salads or bowls.

Grilled Lemon Herb Shrimp:

- In a bowl, combine lemon juice, lemon zest, olive oil, minced garlic, chopped parsley, chopped dill, salt, and pepper to make the marinade.

- Add the peeled and deveined shrimp to the marinade. Toss to coat the shrimp evenly.
- Cover and refrigerate for 15-30 minutes to allow the flavors to meld together.
- Preheat the grill to medium-high heat.
- Thread the marinated shrimp onto skewers, if using.
- Grill the shrimp for 2-3 minutes on each side until pink and opaque.
- Remove from the grill and serve the grilled lemon herb shrimp as a standalone dish or as a delicious addition to salads or pasta.

## Nutritional Information:

The nutritional information for the sustainable seafood and fish recipes may vary based on the specific ingredients used. Please refer to the individual ingredients' nutritional labels for accurate information.

## Lean Poultry and Meat Options

**Description**:

Savor the flavors of lean poultry and meat with these delicious and nutritious recipes. From grilled chicken to roasted turkey, these options provide a good source of high-quality protein while minimizing saturated fat. Enjoy the lean cuts of meat and poultry along with a variety of wholesome ingredients for a well-balanced and satisfying meal.

**Ingredients**:

Grilled Lemon Herb Chicken:

- 4 boneless, skinless chicken breasts
- Juice and zest of 2 lemons
- 3 tablespoons olive oil
- 2 cloves of garlic, minced
- 1 tablespoon chopped fresh rosemary
- 1 tablespoon chopped fresh thyme
- Salt and pepper to taste

Roasted Turkey Tenderloin with Maple Glaze:

- 1 turkey tenderloin
- 2 tablespoons maple syrup
- 2 tablespoons Dijon mustard
- 1 tablespoon olive oil
- 1 teaspoon dried sage
- ½ teaspoon garlic powder
- Salt and pepper to taste

**Instructions**:

Grilled Lemon Herb Chicken:

- In a bowl, combine lemon juice, lemon zest, olive oil, minced garlic, chopped rosemary, chopped thyme, salt, and pepper to make the marinade.
- Add the chicken breasts to the marinade, ensuring they are evenly coated.

- Cover and refrigerate for 30 minutes to 1 hour to allow the flavors to infuse the chicken.
- Preheat the grill to medium-high heat.
- Remove the chicken breasts from the marinade, allowing any excess marinade to drip off.
- Grill the chicken breasts for 6-8 minutes on each side until cooked through and the internal temperature reaches 165°F (74°C).
- Remove from the grill and let them rest for a few minutes before serving.
- Slice the grilled lemon herb chicken and serve as a main dish or in salads, wraps, or sandwiches.

Roasted Turkey Tenderloin with Maple Glaze:

- Preheat the oven to 375°F (190°C).
- In a small bowl, whisk together maple syrup, Dijon mustard, olive oil, dried sage, garlic powder, salt, and pepper to make the glaze.
- Place the turkey tenderloin on a baking sheet lined with parchment paper or foil.
- Brush the glaze over the turkey tenderloin, coating it evenly.
- Roast the turkey tenderloin in the preheated oven for 20-25 minutes or until the internal temperature reaches 165°F (74°C).
- Remove from the oven and let it rest for a few minutes before slicing.
- Serve the roasted turkey tenderloin with maple glaze as a centerpiece for a delicious and lean poultry option.

**Nutritional Information:**

The nutritional information for the lean poultry and meat options may vary based on the specific ingredients used. Please refer to the individual ingredients' nutritional labels for accurate information.

# CONCLUSION

In conclusion, "Lean and Green: A Cookbook for Sustainable Living" not only offers a delectable collection of recipes but also serves as a guide for embracing a healthier and more eco-friendly lifestyle. Throughout this book, we have explored the powerful combination of lean eating and sustainable practices, highlighting the numerous benefits they bring to our well-being and the planet.

By incorporating the principles of lean cooking, we have discovered how to optimize nutrition while reducing waste and unnecessary consumption. From sourcing local and organic ingredients to utilizing innovative cooking techniques that preserve nutrients, we have unlocked the secrets to preparing delicious meals that nourish our bodies and promote overall wellness.

Furthermore, our journey into the realm of green living has revealed how small, conscious choices can have a profound impact on the environment. We have delved into sustainable practices such as reducing food waste, composting, and embracing plant-based alternatives, recognizing the positive influence these choices have on climate change, biodiversity, and the future of our planet.

As we conclude our culinary expedition, let us remember that "Lean and Green" is not just a cookbook—it is a call to action. Each recipe within these pages represents an opportunity to make a difference in our lives and the world around us. By adopting the principles of lean and green cooking, we can forge a path towards a healthier, more sustainable future for ourselves, our communities, and generations to come.

May the recipes and knowledge shared within this book inspire you to explore new culinary horizons, ignite your creativity in the kitchen, and empower you to make informed choices that support both your well-being and the health of our planet. Together, let us savor the joy of nourishing ourselves and the world, one delicious, sustainable meal at a time.

www.ingramcontent.com/pod-product-compliance
Lightning Source LLC
Chambersburg PA
CBHW070045260726

48658CB00002B/743